Homemade Lotion Recipes Free of Toxic Ingredients

Proven Recipes for Natural Lotion

Table of Contents

Introduction

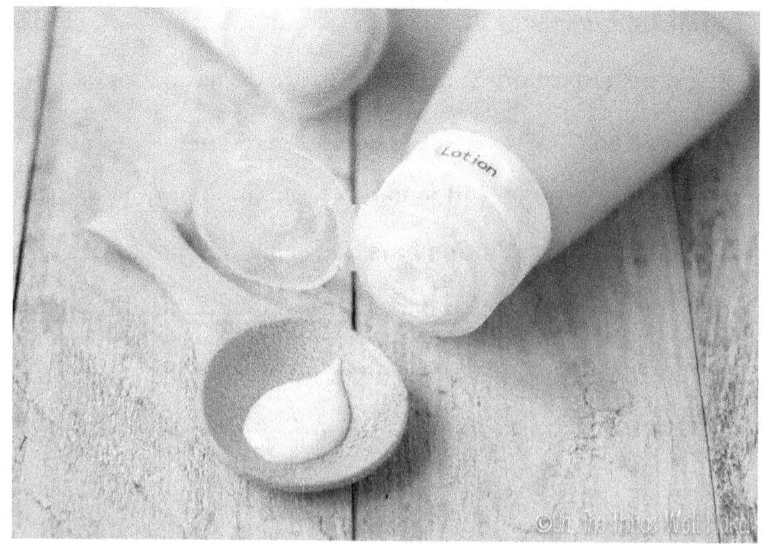

Are you tired of those toxic products and look for the real thing? Our skin is the largest organ. When you apply a lotion with toxic ingredients, they will all be absorbed into the bloodstream. Accumulation of toxins can lead to many health problems, so it is better to avoid ingredients such as parabens, mineral oils, and silicone.

The Homemade Lotion Recipes will teach you how to make natural lotions from scratch. Using affordable ingredients such as essential oils, natural oils, and beeswax, you can prepare the best skincare products.

You can find recipes for:

- Collagen boosting lotion
- Moisturizing glycerine lotion
- Easy eczema lotion
- Pain-relieving dandelion lotion
- Honey and grapefruit body lotion
- Rich chocolate body lotion
- After-sun care lotion
- Chamomile lotion for sensitive skin
- And many other easy lotion recipes!

I invite you to check these easy recipes and become a pro in making lotions!

Collagen boosting lotion

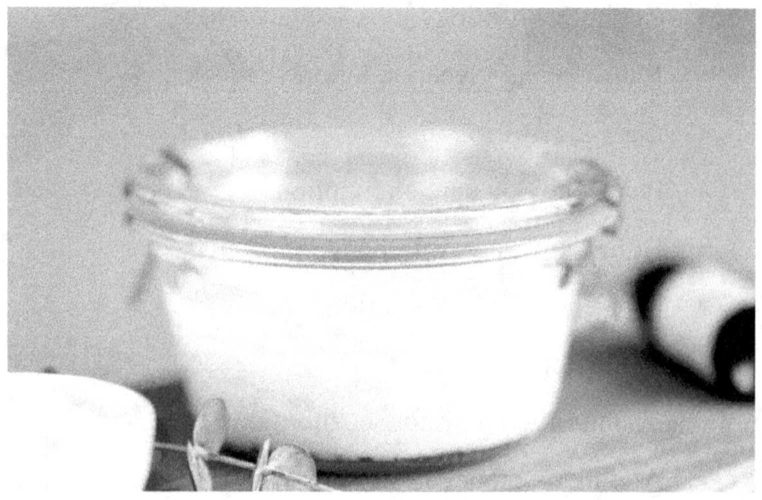

Are you looking for a natural lotion recipe that will stimulate the skin to produce collagen? This recipe is the perfect one. Collagen is known as the protein that helps the skin look younger. This natural lotion is ideal for your face and body. It isn't heavy and won't leave any greasy marks.

Ingredients:

- ¼ cup natural aloe vera gel
- 2 tablespoon grapeseed oil
- ½ cup shea butter

Instructions:

1. In a large bowl, add shea butter and grapeseed oil.

2. Whip on low until it becomes creamy. Scrape down the sides.

3. Add in the aloe vera gel.

4. Slowly increase the speed to high. Continue to mix until fluffy. Scrape down from the sides.

5. Add into a dry and clean jar.

Moisturizing glycerine lotion

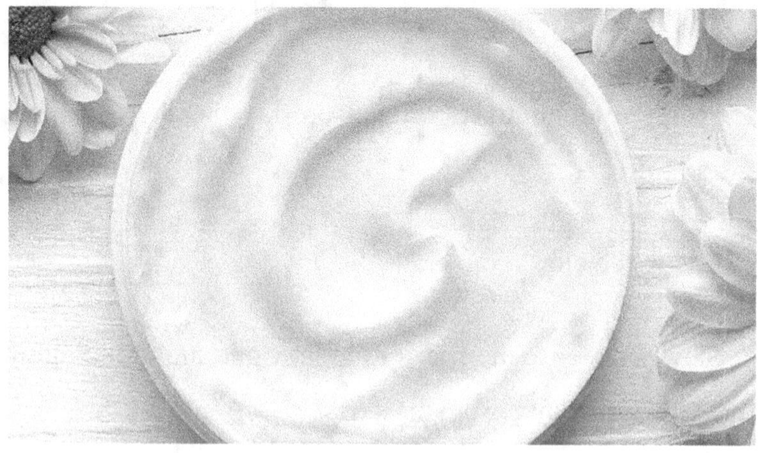

Are you looking for a highly moisturizing lotion that won't leave greasy traces? This recipe has one secret ingredient: glycerin. It is a natural ingredient that will make your skin silky smooth and hydrated. The recipe is quite simple so that anyone can do it even at home. The formula is convenient for dry and sensitive skin but will work with oily skin too.

Ingredients:

- 1.5 oz Emulsifying Wax
- 8 oz Glycerin
- 4.5 oz Coconut Oil
- 16 oz Distilled Water

Instructions:

Add coconut oil and wax in a bowl. Melt in a double boiler on the stove.

Add water and glycerin. Make sure that you use only distilled water so that your lotion will last longer. Mix well.

Pour into clean and dry jars. When the weather is hot, keep your lotion in the fridge.

Baby lotion

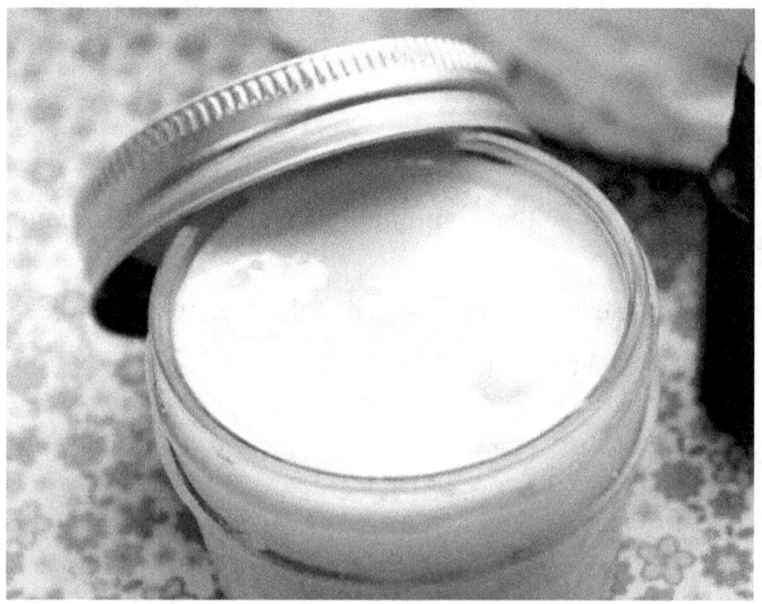

Are you looking for a gentle lotion recipe that is suitable for a baby? It is always better to avoid exposing your baby to chemicals. This recipe will show you how to prepare a DIY lotion. It is completely natural, so you won't have to worry about anything. The formula will offer proper care for the baby's gentle skin.

Ingredients:

- 1/2 cup of shea butter
- 1 tablespoon of Sweet Almond oil

- 1/4 cup coconut oil

- 1 tablespoon of Aloe Vera gel

- 5 drops Lavender essential oil

- 5 drops of Cedarwood essential oil

Instructions:

1. Add the shea butter into a large mixing bowl. Whip it on high for a minute, until no lumps remain.

2. Add coconut oil, aloe vera gel, and almond oil. Whip for 30 seconds on high.

3. Scrape down the sides. Lower the speed to medium and add the essential oils.

4. When it is all combined, transfer to a dry and clean jar.

Easy eczema lotion

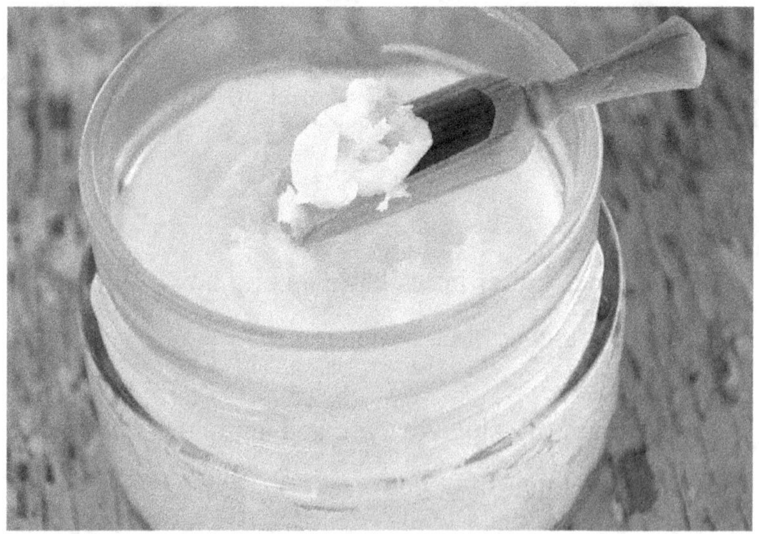

Eczema can be a really annoying issue. The best solution is to apply natural and rich lotion to nourish the skin. Here is a recipe that you can whip up in your kitchen easily. It has natural ingredients that will battle the flakiness. Apply three times a day to relieve the dryness.

Ingredients:

- 1/2 cup chamomile infused coconut oil
- 1/2 cup shea butter
- 1 tablespoon olive oil
- 1/4 cup oatmeal

- 1 tablespoon honey

Instructions:

1. Put the oatmeal in a blender. Blend until ground to a fine powder.

2. In a microwave-safe bowl place the shea butter and coconut oil. Microwave for 30 seconds, until they are melted.

3. Remove and add honey and olive oil. Mix well.

4. When the mixture starts to harden, add in the ground oatmeal. Mix well

5. Transfer to clean 4 oz jar. Store it and remember to stir it occasionally.

Non-greasy and fast-absorbing lotion

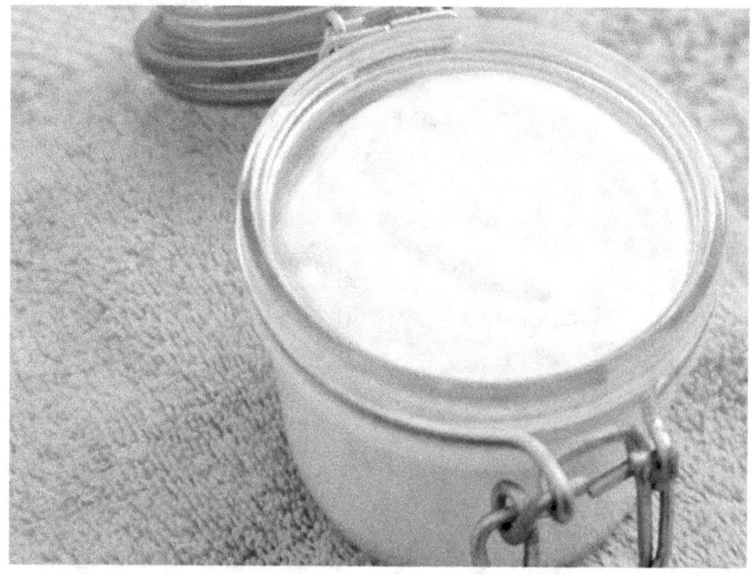

During the summer, your skin won't need any heavy lotions. This is the time when light formulas step in. This non-greasy lotion has carefully picked ingredients that won't leave greasy traces behind. Jojoba oil and aloe vera are known for their fast-absorbing ability.

They will be absorbed fast and will feed your skin with the needed nutrients.

Ingredients:

- 1/2 tablespoon raw Shea butter

- 1/2 cup aloe vera gel

- 1/2 tablespoon Argan oil

- 1/2 cup jojoba oil

- 10-12 drops mint essential oil

- 1 and 1/2 tablespoon beeswax pellets

Instructions:

1. Start by Create a double-boiler. Use a small saucepan and a medium heat-proof bowl. Bring water in the saucepan to boil.

2. In the bowl, add Shea butter and beeswax. Add the bowl on top of the saucepan. Mix them until they melt.

3. Add in the rest of the ingredients. Stir occasionally. The mixture will need from 5 to 10 minutes to be melted and well combined.

4. Remove the bowl carefully using oven mitts. Allow it to cool for 30-45 minutes, but don't let it get too hard.

5. Use a hand mixer to whip it until you reach a lotion-like consistency. Pour to a dry and clean jar or another glass container.

Pain-relieving dandelion lotion

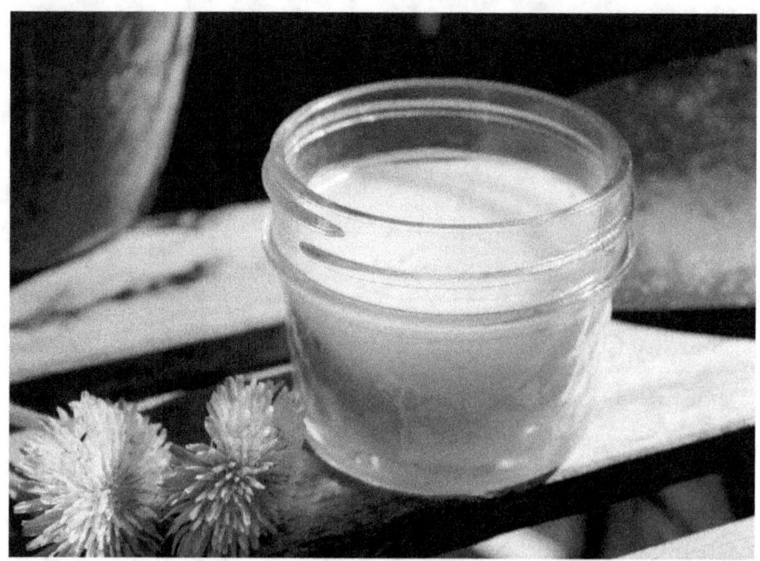

Dandelions have natural pain-relieving properties. This makes the herb the best choice for your lotion. Another key ingredient is magnesium. In modern times, our bodies lack magnesium. When you apply it on the skin, it will be adequately absorbed. The lotion will release the sore muscles and relieve the pain.

Ingredients:

- 3 teaspoon emulsifying wax
- 2 tablespoon dandelion-infused oil
- 5 teaspoon distilled water

- 2 tablespoon magnesium oil

- 2 to 3 drops lavender essential oil

- 1 tablespoon aloe vera gel

- preservative of choice

Instructions:

1. Pour the dandelion-infused oil and emulsifying wax into a clean tin can.

2. Put magnesium oil, water, and aloe vera gel into a second tin can.

3. Add about two inches of water in a saucepan. Set over medium-low heat.

4. Once the content in the first can is melted, transfer it into a bowl together with the content from the second tin.

5. Use a whisk to mix them well. Let it cool for 5 minutes, while occasionally mixing.

6. Add in essential oil and mix. Add the preservative as well.

7. Pour into a clean container. The mixture will get thicker in the next 24 hours.

Honey and grapefruit body lotion

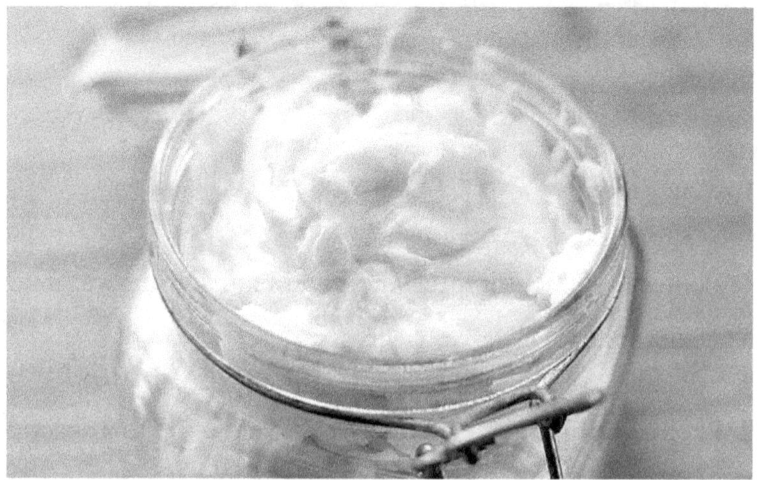

This recipe features a rich and creamy lotion that has a fresh citrus scent. The natural essential oil gives that gentle fragrance, which is better than any store-bought lotion. The addition of honey will nourish your skin and protect it.

Ingredients:

- 1.5 tablespoons honey
- 2 tablespoons coconut oil
- 1.5 tablespoons beeswax
- 1 tablespoon shea butter
- 1 tablespoon almond oil
- 20 drops grapefruit essential oil

Instructions:

1. Place all of your ingredients in a double boiler. Het over medium. Let all of the ingredients melt for about 15 minutes and whisk occasionally.

2. Leave for 1 to 2 minutes. Add in essential oil drops and mix again.

3. Let it harden for more than 6 hours.

4. Once hardened, whip with a hand mixer. 2 to 3 minutes are enough for the mixture to get fluffy. Transfer to a clean and dry container.

Rich chocolate body lotion

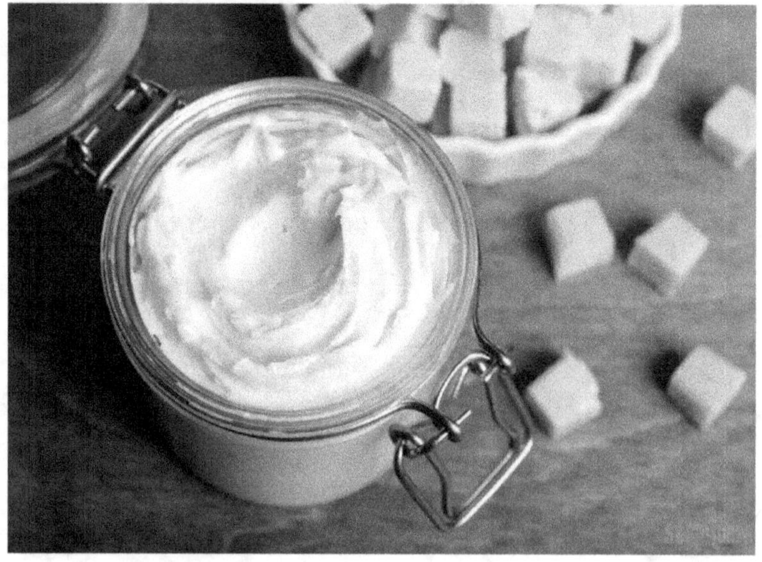

Do you love the smell of chocolate? Now, you can have it on your body. This recipe will show you how to make soothing and rich body lotion with an irresistible chocolate scent. The cacao powder will bring scent as well as additional benefits. It is a well-known antioxidant, so it will keep your skin protected from free radicals.

Ingredients:

- 1/2 cup coconut oil
- 1 cup of cocoa butter
- 2 tablespoons sweet almond oil

- 1 teaspoon beeswax

- 1 1/2 tablespoons cocoa powder

- 1 tablespoon vanilla extract

Instructions:

1. Melt coconut oil, cocoa butter, beeswax in a double boiler. It will take about 10 minutes.

2. Add the rest ingredients and mix well. Leave in the fridge for one hour.

3. The mixture is ready to be whipped when the top is hardened, but the rest is still liquid.

4. Whip on low, while slowly increasing the speed. It will take about 10 minutes for your lotion to get all fluffy.

5. Transfer to a clean container of your choice.

After-sun care lotion

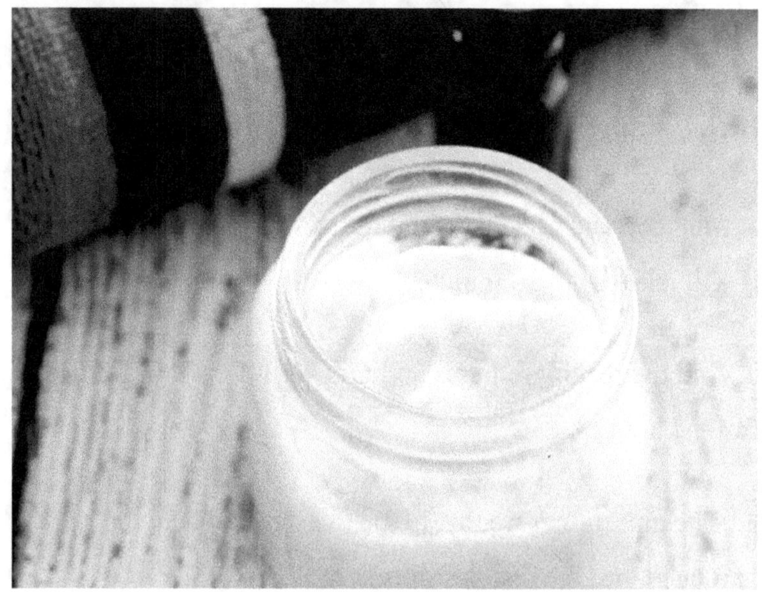

The vacation season comes with one unpleasant problem: sunburns. If you forget to apply your sunscreen, the result can be quite painful. But there is one remedy that you can whip up in your kitchen. This after-sun lotion contains all of the secret ingredients that will speed up the healing process. Aloe vera will cool down the skin, while the natural olive oil will fix the damage.

Ingredients:

- 1 teaspoon Shea butter
- 3 tablespoons calendula infused olive oil with
- 1 tablespoon grated or granulated beeswax
- 1 teaspoon cocoa butter
- 1 tablespoon coconut oil
- 3 tablespoons aloe vera gel
- 15 drops lavender essential oil

Instructions:

1. Put all of the oils, butters, and beeswax in a double-boiler. Set to medium heat. Mix to combine them well.

2. Once melted add in the essential oils. Cool for 5 minutes and add aloe vera gel. Mix well until combined.

3. Store in clean containers. Apply a generous amount on the burnt skin.

Chamomile lotion for sensitive skin

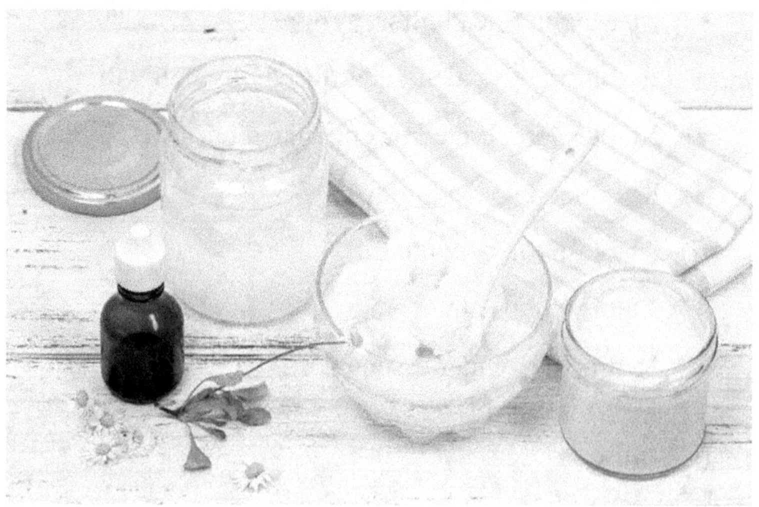

This lotion recipe is suitable for sensitive skin. Chamomile is well-known for its calming abilities. And it is highly recommended for people with sensitive skin. The avocado butter will make the skin soft and smooth.

Ingredients:

- 1 tablespoon avocado butter
- 1 tablespoon chamomile infused avocado oil
- 6 tablespoons distilled water
- 1 tablespoon emulsifying wax NF
- nature-derived preservative

Instructions:

1. Add oil, butter and emulsifying wax in a heatproof jar.

2. Add the water in a second jar.

3. Place both jars in a saucepan with water. Turn to medium-low heat.

4. Let the first mixture melt for 10 minutes. Remove

5. Pour the content of both jars in a bowl. Mix for 30 seconds. Let it cool for 5 minutes but mix occasionally. Add the preservative Leave it for a few hours to cool completely, with occasional stirring.

6. Transfer to clean jar and use when needed.

Body lotion with rose and hibiscus

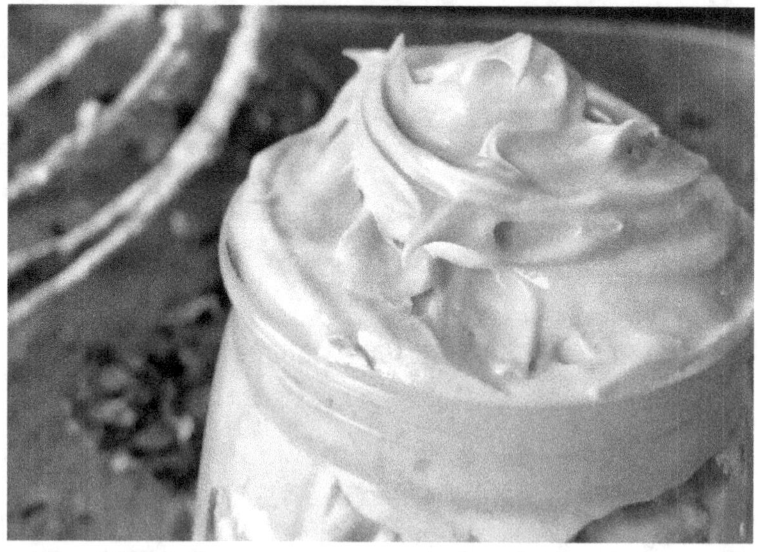

This homemade lotion recipe can make the perfect gift for someone. That sweet rose scent will amaze every lady. The carefully picked ingredients make this lotion the right choice for skincare. It has a well-balanced mix of natural oils that does wonders to the skin.

Ingredients:

- 1 Cup Coconut Oil
- 1 teaspoon Almond Oil
- 8 drops Rose Essential Oil
- Brewed Hibiscus Tea

Instructions:

1. Add softened coconut oil and almond oil into a bowl.

2. Add a few drops of tea and the rose essential oil. This will give color and smell to your lotion.

3. Mix with mixer until it becomes fluffy and airy. It will take you around 10 minutes.

4. Transfer to a clean and dry jar.

Magnesium lotion for sore muscles

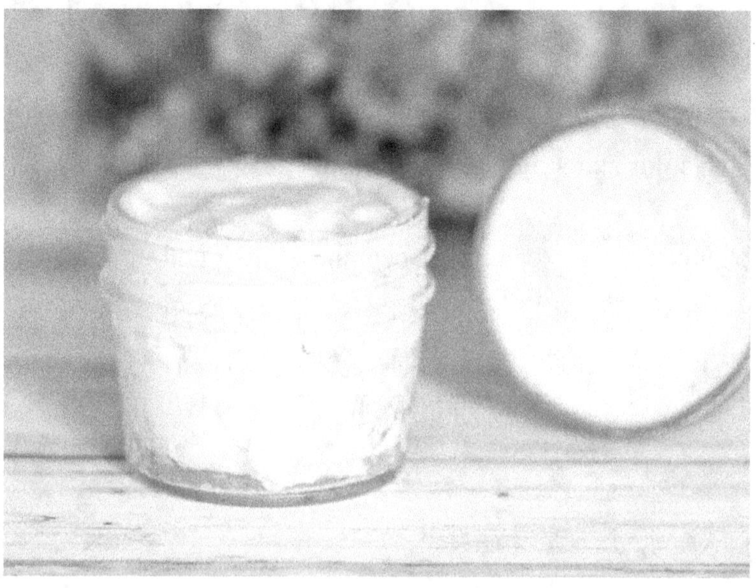

Are you looking for a lotion that will relieve the pain from sore muscles? This recipe will show you how to prepare your own. It uses magnesium oil, which can be made if you mix magnesium flakes and water. For 1/2 cup magnesium oil, you will need ½ cup flakes and 3 tablespoons of hot water.

Ingredients:

- 1/4 cup coconut oil
- 5 grams beeswax
- 1/2 cup magnesium oil
- 7 tablespoons raw shea butter

- tablespoon arrowroot powder

- Few drops geranium essential oil

Instructions:

1. Add the coconut oil, beeswax, and shea butter in a heatproof jar. Place it in a saucepan with 3 inches of water. Set it to medium heat. Turn off when the water comes to simmer.

2. Stir the oils so that they combine when melted. Once everything is nicely melted, remove. Let it cool until it looks cloudy.

3. Use an immersion blender or a hand mixer to blend it well.

4. Add the magnesium oil slowly while mixing. Blend until everything is combined.

5. Add powder and essential oils and mix again.

6. Transfer to clean jars and use according to your needs.

After-shave lotion

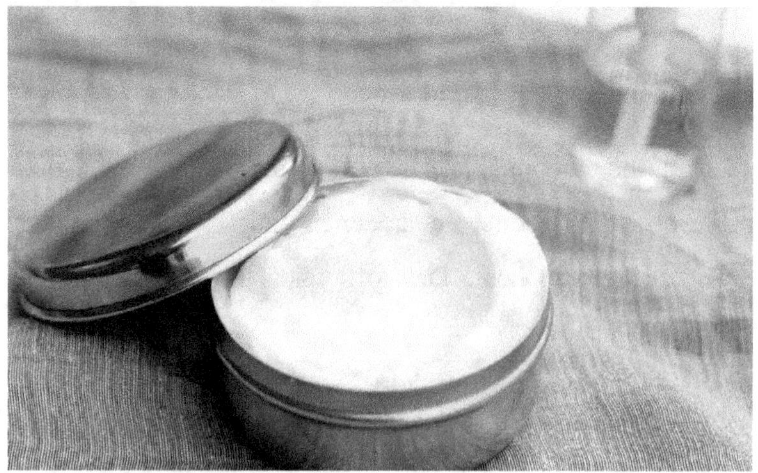

Here you have an easy recipe for after-shave lotion, both suitable for women and men. It soothes the skin and calms the trauma caused by the razor. The aloe vera will calm any irritations, while the witch hazel is known as an excellent toner.

Ingredients:

- 1/2 tablespoon coconut oil
- 1/4 teaspoon witch hazel
- 1/2 tablespoon aloe vera gel

Instructions:

1. Place the ingredients in a bowl.

2. Mix well until they are well combined.

3. Transfer to a clean container of your choice. Use after shaving. You don't need to rinse off this homemade lotion.

Pumpkin spice lotion

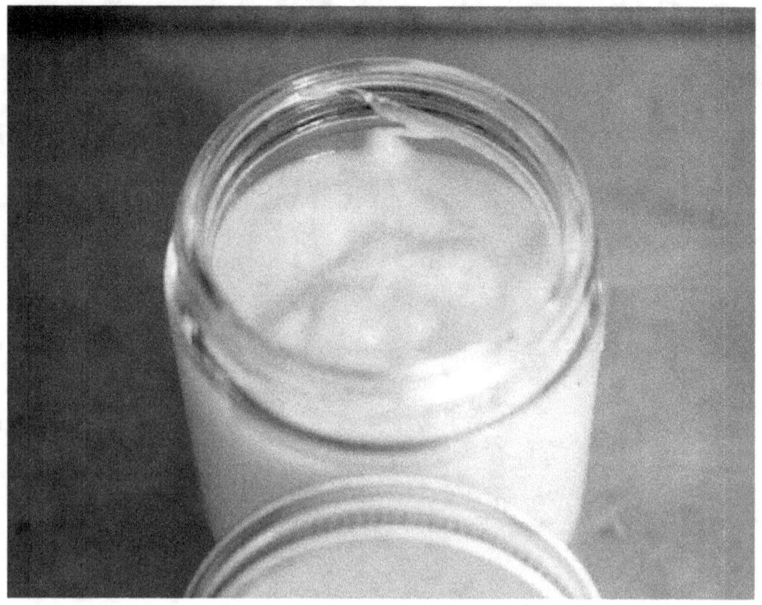

This is a lotion recipe that is perfect for winter and fall. We all love the cozy scent of pumpkin spice, so this is an excellent way to enjoy it. The lotion will have a beautiful color because of the addition of paprika. Plus, it will have an incredible smell because of the essential oils.

Ingredients:

- 2 tablespoons almond oil
- 1/4 cup cocoa butter
- 1/8-1/4 teaspoon paprika

- 2 tablespoons coconut oil

- 1 teaspoon beeswax

- 5 drops nutmeg essential oil

- 10 drops cinnamon essential oil

- 7 drops ginger essential oil

- 2 drops clove essential oil

- 2 drops allspice essential oil

Instructions:

1. Mix the cocoa butter, coconut oil, almond oil, and beeswax in a pot. Put it over a larger pot with boiling water. Stir until melted and well combined.

2. Add paprika and mix well. Leave for 10 minutes. Remove paprika that isn't dissolved.

3. Put in the fridge. Remove before it gets completely solid.

4. Add all of the essential oils. Whip for one minute with a hand mixer, starting from low and slowly increasing to high.

5. Transfer to clean container.

Texas Cedarwood lotion recipe

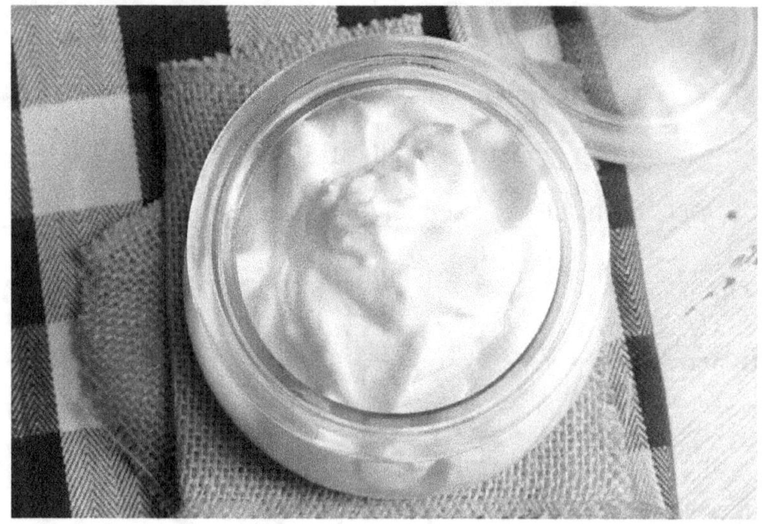

Texas cedarwood essential oil has so many benefits. It is used for preventing dry scalp, headaches, and colds. This would make it the perfect ingredient for a lotion. This recipe will show you how to make it. The perfect amount of essential oils is crucial, so don't miss this one!

Ingredients:

- 1 ½ ounce coconut oil
- 6 ounces aloe vera gel
- 10 drops Texas cedarwood essential oil
- 1 teaspoon vitamin E oil

Instructions:

1. Pour the aloe vera gel and coconut oil in a mixing bowl. Beat with an electric mixer for 3 minutes.

2. Add in the remaining oils. Continue to beat on low.

3. When you are done, store it into a clean container. Alternatively, you can put it in a clean plastic bag and pipe it into a dispenser bottle. This way, you can easily get the desired amount without getting your fingers into the container.

Mango body lotion

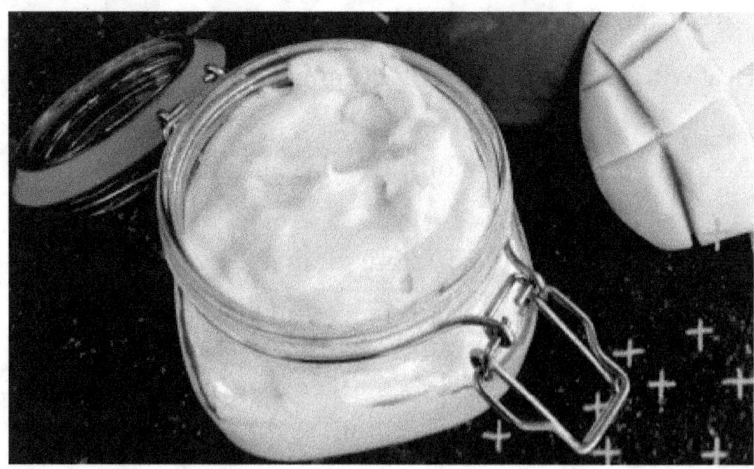

Mango butter is well known for its nourishing properties. As soon as you come out of the shower, you would want to apply this excellent smelling lotion to your body. This whipped body lotion is perfect for your dry skin. You can use it instead of massage oil too.

Ingredients:

- 1 1/3 tablespoon cocoa butter
- 1 1/3 tablespoon mango butter
- 2 tablespoons shea butter
- 1 1/3 tablespoon apricot kernel oil
- 2 tablespoons coconut oil

- 20 drops citrus essential oil: 5 lemon, 5 lime, 5 sweet orange, 5 pink grapefruit

Instructions:

1. Add the coconut, apricot oils and butters into a double boiler. Mix so that everything is well combined when melted.

2. Prepare a cold bath. In a large bowl, put water and ice. Place the pot with the mixture on top of that, so that it chills more quickly.

3. When the mixture has cooled down slightly, start to whip using a hand mixer. Whip until you reach a nice fluffy consistency.

4. Transfer to a clean and dry container. You can use it within a few months.

Gingerbread body lotion recipe

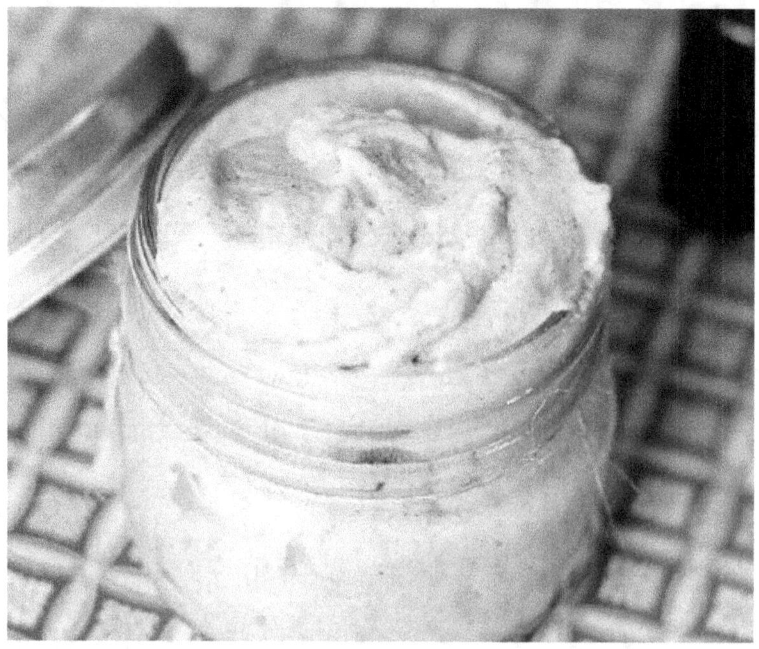

As soon as the cold weather comes, it is time for a rich and nourishing body lotion. This one has the specific smell of gingerbread. It reminds us of holidays and coziness. The unusual secret ingredient is ginger oil. Not only that it smells divine, but it has antioxidant properties. It will improve skin elasticity and tone. Cinnamon essential oil is known for the antibacterial properties so that it will prevent acne.

Ingredients:

- ½ cup Shea butter
- ½ cup of coconut oil
- 1 T. ground ginger
- 1 teaspoon cinnamon
- 5 drops ginger essential oil
- 5 drops cinnamon essential oil
- 1 teaspoon vanilla extract

Instructions:

1. In a saucepan over medium heat, melt the coconut oil and shea butter. Make sure that you mix regularly.

2. Pour into a mixing bowl. Leave it in the fridge for 15 minutes.

3. Next, add the spices, essential oils, and vanilla extract. Whip with a hand mixer about 5 minutes on high.

4. Transfer to a clean sealed container.

Peppermint body lotion

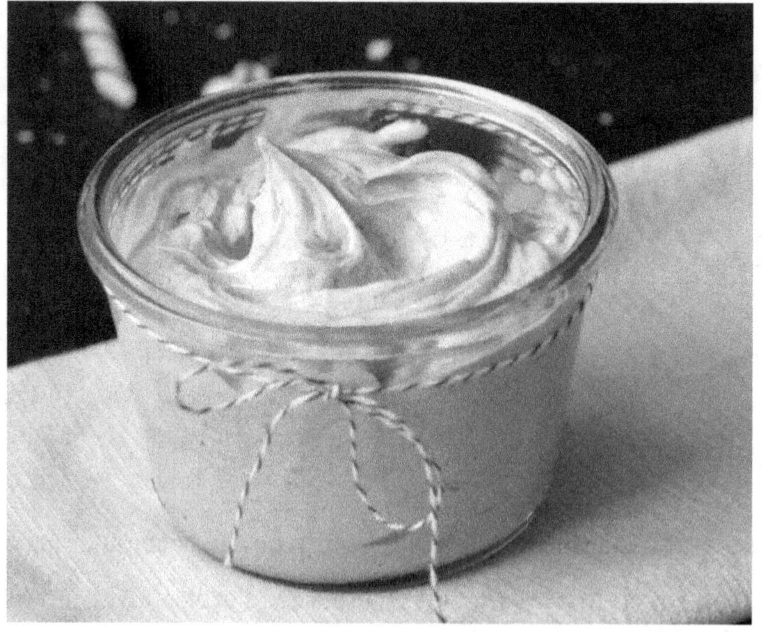

This is another boy lotion recipe inspired by the holidays. This is an excellent lotion that you can whip up for the winter. With its fantastic smell and nourishing ingredients, it will make sure that your skin stays hydrated. But, feel free to use it all year round.

Ingredients:

- 2 tablespoons Coconut Oil
- 1/4 cup Shea Butter
- 1 teaspoon Vitamin E

- 1/2 teaspoons. beetroot powder
- 15- 20 drops peppermint essential oil

Instructions:

1. Chop the shea butter to smaller pieces. Transfer to a microwave-safe bowl. Put it for 30 seconds in the micro. Take it out and stir. Repeat until melted.

2. Add the melted butter into a mixing bowl. Whip in the rest of the oils.

3. Put the mixing bowl in the fridge for 15 minutes.

4. Remove and whip until fluffy. Add in the beetroot powder while whipping. It will give a nice pink color to your body lotion.

5. Put into a clean container and use it accordingly.

Cooling lotion for legs and feet

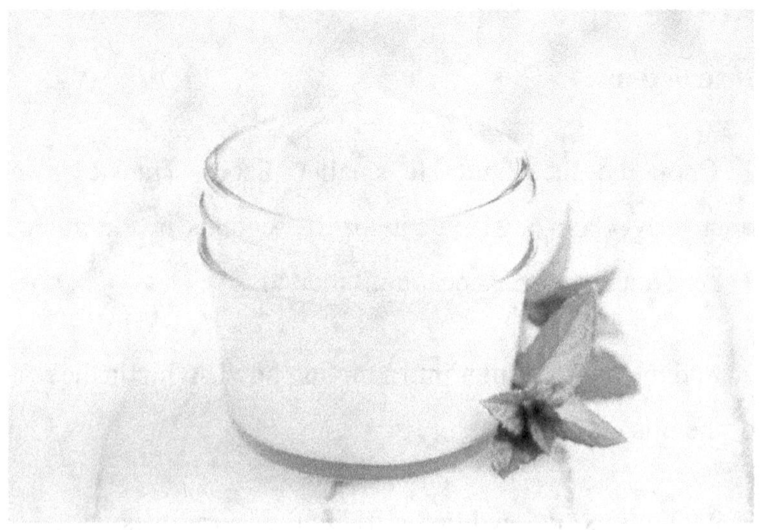

Need something to relieve the pain after a long day of walking or standing? This cooling lotion is excellent for tired legs and feet. Also, it is a great way to relieve the pain once you have removed the high heels. It also has a carefully picked mix of essential oils that remove bad odors. The nourishing butters will leave your skin silky soft, which is one more reason why you should whip up this lotion.

Ingredients:

- ¼ cup mango butter
- ¼ cup virgin coconut oil
- 1 teaspoon vitamin e oil

- 15 drops tea tree oil
- 15 drops peppermint oil
- 5 drops eucalyptus oil

Instructions:

1. Melt coconut oils and mango butter over a double boiler. Remove once it is melted and be careful not to overheat.

2. Add in essential oils and vitamin e. Stir well.

3. Put in the fridge for a few minutes. The mixture should come to room temperature.

4. Transfer to a mixing bowl and whip using a mixer. Finish when the color is lighter, and texture is creamy.

5. Transfer to a clean container. Your homemade lotion will last for three months.

Baby lotion recipe

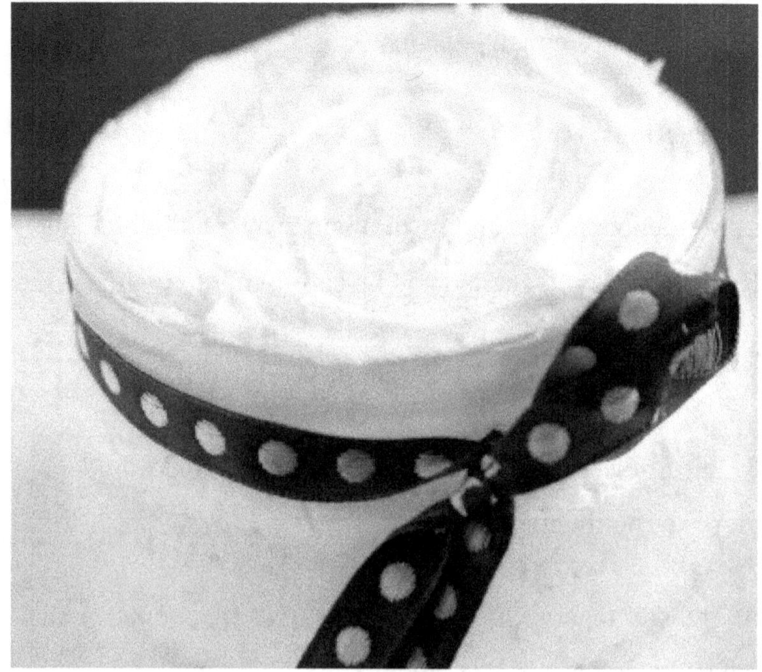

Baby skin needs natural and toxin-free lotions. When you don't want those store-bought versions full of preservatives and mineral oils, you can turn to this recipe. It isn't greasy but will provide the baby skin with the needed moisture.

Ingredients:

- 1/2 cup aloe vera gel
- 1/2 cup coconut oil
- Essential oil – several drops (optional)

Instructions:

1. Melt the coconut oil over hot water. Add it into your blender, or you can use even a food processor for this recipe.

2. Add in the cold aloe vera gel. Add a few drops of your essential oils.

3. Blend until well combined. Transfer to a clean container and store it in the fridge or at room temperature. If your home is warm, then the lotion will be runny so you can place it in the fridge.

Anti-aging body lotion recipe

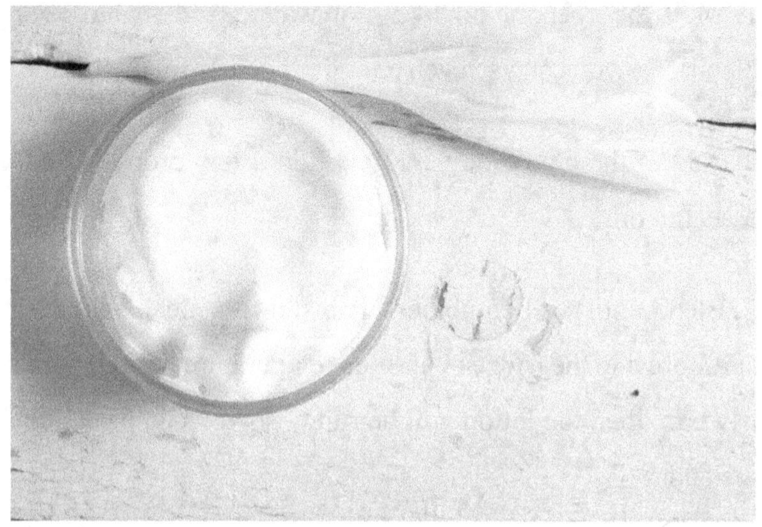

Aging is a natural body process. As the years pass, your skin will get less elastic, and wrinkles will appear. The right skincare will slow down the natural process of aging. The sun can damage your skin, so it is good to use SPF all year round. This body lotion has everything needed to slow down the aging. It has natural SPF to protect your skin, as well as antioxidants, Vitamin A, and Vitamin E to moisturize.

Ingredients:

- 2 ½ Tablespoons Apricot Kernel Oil
- ½ cup Shea Butter
- 1 teaspoon Nano Zinc Oxide

- 2-½ Tablespoons Argan Oil

- 5 drops Lavender Essential Oil

- 5 drops Frankincense Essential Oil

- 5 drops of Geranium Essential Oil

- 5 drops Carrot Seed Essential Oil

Instructions:

1. Add the shea butter in a mixing bowl. Whip with a mixer until creamy.

2. Slowly add apricot and argan oil while still mixing.

3. Remove the mixer. Add in the Nano Zinc Oxide and mix with a spoon.

4. Add the essential oils and whip with mixer again. Stop when everything is well combined and fluffy.

5. Transfer to a clean container. When using, massage the lotion into your skin so that it won't leave white traces.

Hot chocolate lotion bar

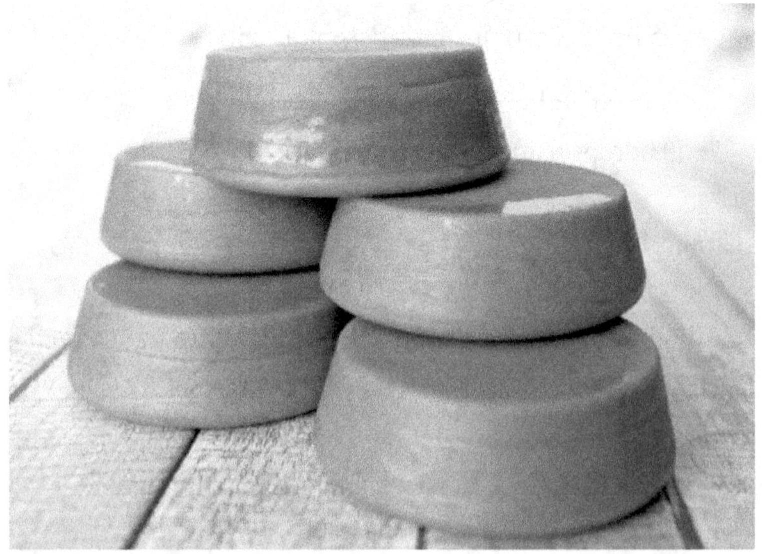

Do you love to have a cup of hot chocolate? Why not have it on your skin too? This body lotion smells like your favorite drink in winter. The best thing is that it is made of ingredients that your skin will absolutely love.

Ingredients:

- 1/4 cup Cocoa Butter
- 1/2 cup Beeswax
- 1 Teaspoon Cocoa Powder
- 1 tablespoon. Avocado Oil
- 2 tablespoons. Almond Oil

- 1/2 teaspoon vitamin e oil

- 50 drops (approx. 1/2 tsp) vanilla essential oil

Instructions:

1. Melt your cocoa butter and beeswax using a double boiler. Remove when melted.

2. Add almond and avocado oils.

3. Whisk in the cocoa powder.

4. Next, add vanilla essential oil and vitamin e oil. Mix well.

5. Pour into silicone molds of your choice. Wait for them to harden before you remove them.

Vanilla lotion bar

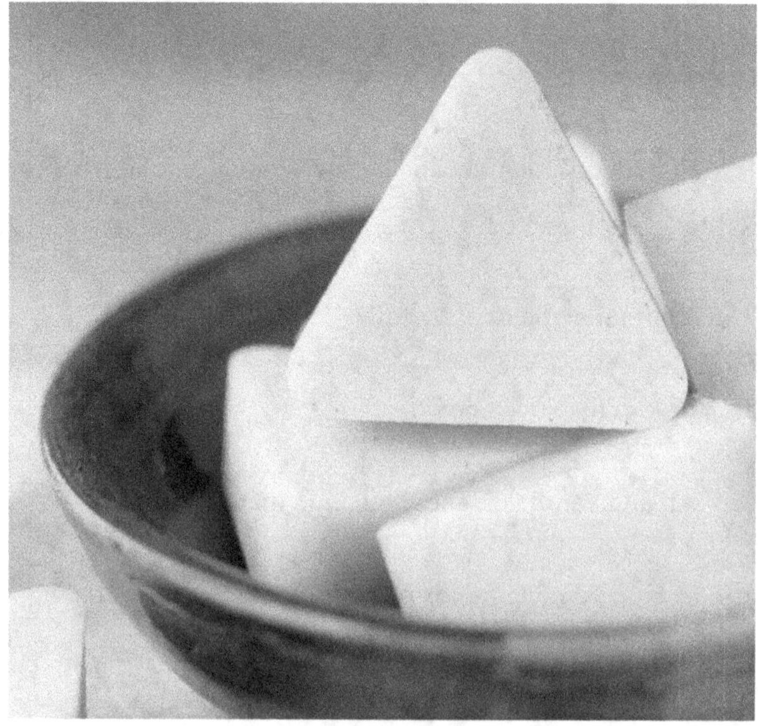

Vanilla is an all-time favorite smell. With these homemade lotion bars, your skin will smell like the pure and sweet vanilla beans. The best thing is that it is made of nourishing oils, which are perfect for winter skincare. The bar shape makes the process of application much easier.

Ingredients:

- 2 tablespoons coconut oil
- 2 ounces cocoa butter
- 10 drops vanilla essential oil

Instructions:

1. Melt cocoa butter and coconut oil over medium heat in a small pot. Stir the mixture constantly until they melt and watch out so that they don't overheat.

2. Remove from heat once melted. Add in the vanilla essential oil and stir well until combined.

3. Pour the mixture in your preferred silicone molds. Put the mold in the fridge for 2 hours, or until your bars harden.

Apple lotion bars

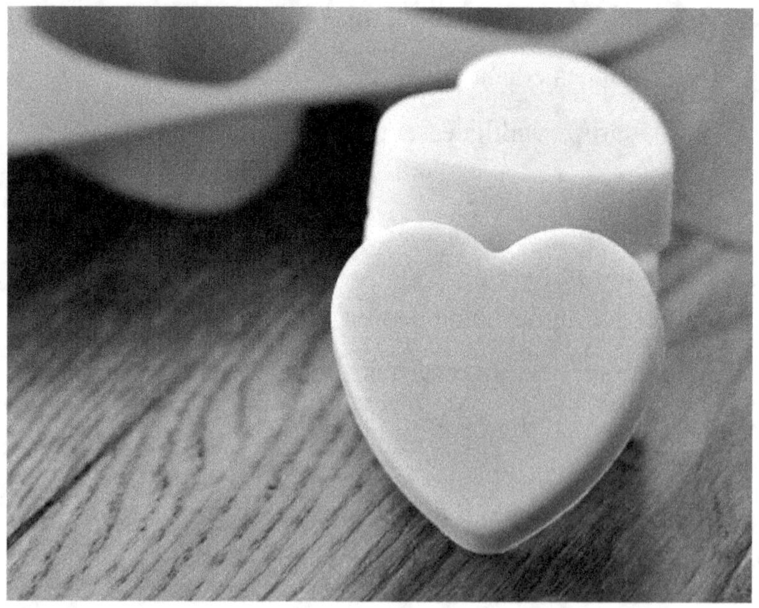

Apple is one of the favorite fall scents. These homemade lotion bars have that specific mild fragrance, perfect for the cold days. The beeswax will protect your skin against drying, once those cold winds start. You can make these in a short time, so let's get to the recipe!

Ingredients:

- 1/3 cup coconut oil
- 1/3 cup beeswax
- 1/3 cup shea butter soap base

- 8-10 drops red soap colorant

- 10-12 drops apple soap fragrance

Instructions:

1. Place shea butter, beeswax pellets, and coconut oil in a heat-safe bowl.

2. Put in the micro on high for 30 seconds, then remove and stir. Place the bowl back for another 30-second interval. Repeat up to three times, or until they have melted.

3. Remove from the microwave once completely melted. Add in the fragrance and colorant. Mix well.

4. Pour the mixture in your silicone molds. Let them chill for 30 minutes, or until completely hardened.

Bug repellent lotion

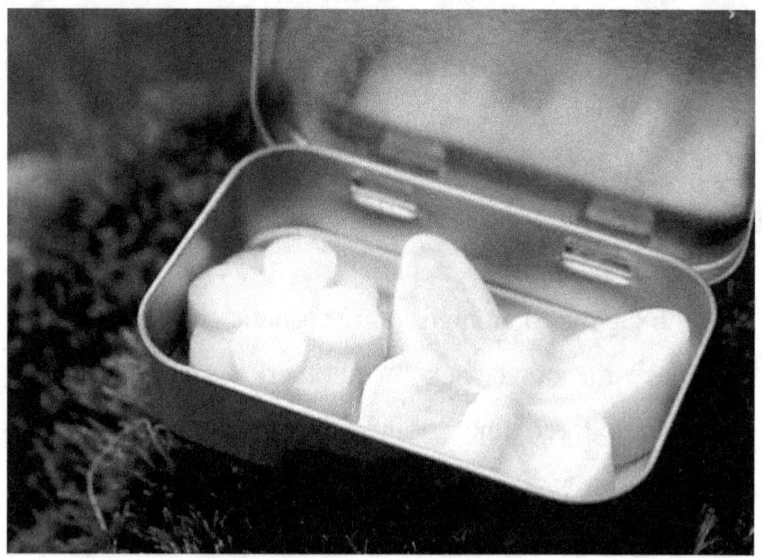

The only thing that we all hate about summer is the bugs. Mosquitoes, flies, and ticks will prevent you from having a great time outdoors. But this lotion recipe is here to save you. With having a few secret ingredients, it will repel the insects away from your skin. Plus, it doesn't have any synthetic fragrances or ingredients.

Ingredients:

- 1/4 cup beeswax
- 1/4 cup mango butter
- 1/2 cup kokum butter

- 2 tablespoons apricot kernel oil

- 1/4 cup babassu oil

- 100 drops lemon eucalyptus essential oil

- 62 drops geranium essential oil

- 1/4 cup arrowroot powder

Instructions:

1. In a bowl, add beeswax, oils, and butter. Melt over a double boiler.

2. Remove from heat when melted.

3. Add in the essential oils and mix well.

4. Add the arrowroot powder and mix until there are no lumps visible.

5. Pour the mixture into silicone molds. Let them chill in the fridge or room temperature.

Massage lotion bar

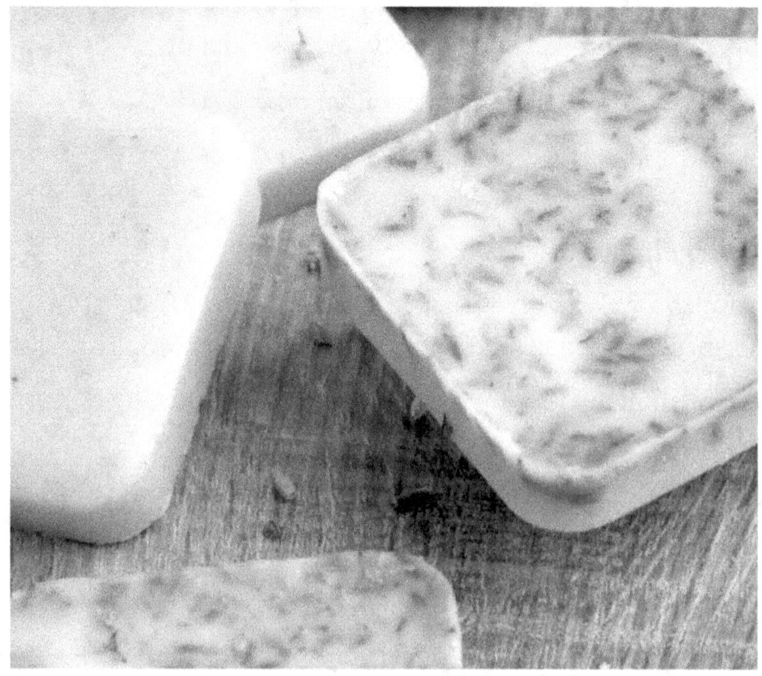

Do you want to enjoy a good massage? You can now do it in the comfort of your own home. These DIY lotion bars will embrace your body with moisturizing oils and fantastic fragrances.

Ingredients:

- 2 oz Beeswax
- 2 oz Deodorized Cocoa Butter
- 2 oz Shea Butter

- 1/2 oz Jojoba Oil

- 1 oz Sweet Almond Oil

- 18 Drops of Lavender Oil

- 18 Drops of Sweet Orange Oil

Instructions:

1. First, start melting the beeswax. Once it is melted, add in the cocoa and shea butter. Mix and melt again.

2. Once everything is well mixed and melted, mix in almond oil and jojoba oil. Add the essential oils too.

3. Pour the mixture in massage bar molds. Let them harden before removing.

Non-greasy summer lotion bar

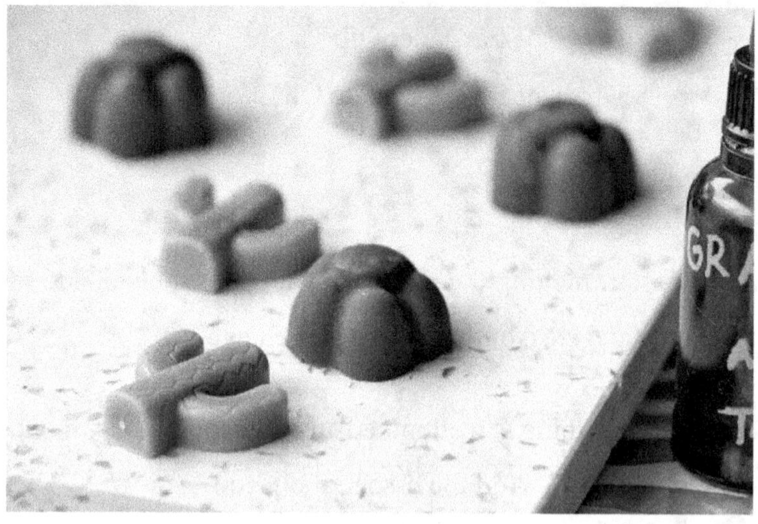

Lotion bars are an absolute favorite for busy people. They are so easy to apply and work wonders for your skin. Place one in a tin box, and you have it ready for traveling. This summer lotion bar is perfect for your vacation. You can slip it in your hand luggage, without worrying about the liquid limits.

Ingredients:

- 1 cup unrefined cocoa butter
- 1 cup beeswax pastilles
- 1 cup extra virgin coconut oil
- 2 tablespoons. extra virgin olive oil

- 4 tablespoons dried rose petals
- 3 tablespoons dried calendula flowers
- 30-40 drops lavender essential oil
- 3 tablespoons dried lavender buds

Instructions:

1. Put calendula, cocoa butter, roses, lavender, and coconut oil in a pan over medium heat. Mix until they are all melted. Keep the temperature to 167 °F for 1-2 hours. Watch out so that the oils don't get hot.

2. Strain out the mixture to remove the herbs.

3. Place the mixture into a clean saucepan. Add the beeswax in.

4. Place the saucepan over medium heat until melted.

5. Pour the completely melted mixture into molds. Let them cool for an hour.

Mosquito repellent lotion bars

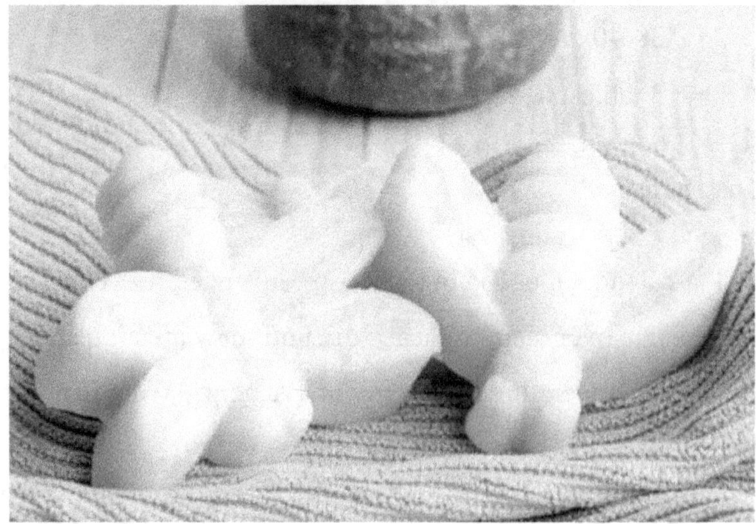

This lotion recipe is perfect for the summer months when the boring mosquitos won't let you enjoy outdoor. The carefully picked combination of essential oils will chase away the insects, leaving your skin with a nice smell. This bar recipe is so convenient for use too.

Ingredients:

- 1 tablespoon beeswax
- 4 tablespoons Shea butter
- 2 tablespoons Coconut oil
- 5 drops lemon essential oil

- 10 drops jojoba oil

- 10 drops citronella Oil

- 20 drops lemongrass essential oil

- 5 drops peppermint essential oil

Instructions:

1. Place all the ingredients in a bowl. Melt over a double boiler. Set temperature to medium.

2. Stir constantly until the ingredients are melted. You shouldn't have any lumps.

3. When the liquid mixture is well combined, pour it into silicone molds of your choice. Let them cool down and harden completely. You can now remove the bars and store them in containers.

Relaxing lavender lotion bars

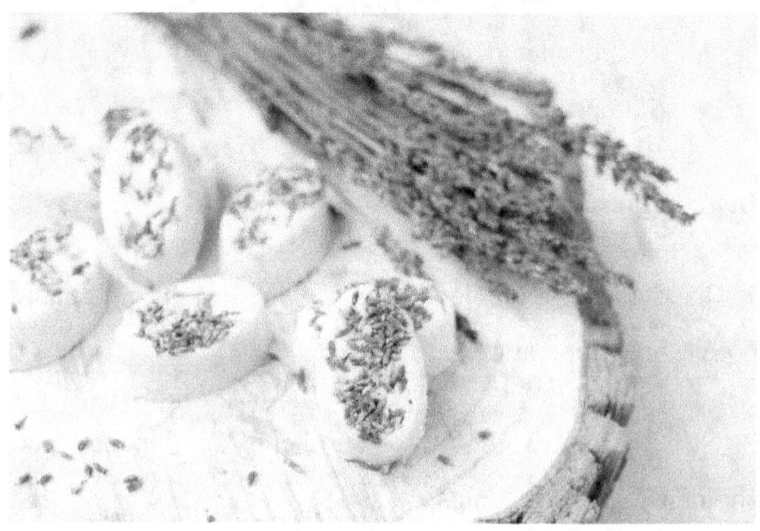

Lavender is known for the ability to relax your body. It also helps in the fight against insomnia. These lotion bars are perfect if you want to get a good night sleep. Rub them onto your hands, so that the body heat will melt the natural oils. Apply all over your body and enjoy the wonderful lavender scent.

Ingredients:

- 1/2 cup shea butter
- 1 cup beeswax
- 1 Cup coconut oil
- 15-20 drops Lavender essential oil

Instructions:

In a small saucepan melt your beeswax and coconut oil. Stir until melted.

Add in the shea butter. Stir until melted.

Remove from the stove. Add the essential oil. Mix well.

Pour the liquid into your silicone molds. Let it cool overnight. Once hardened, you can safely remove your DIY lotion bars.

Lemon and basil lotion bars

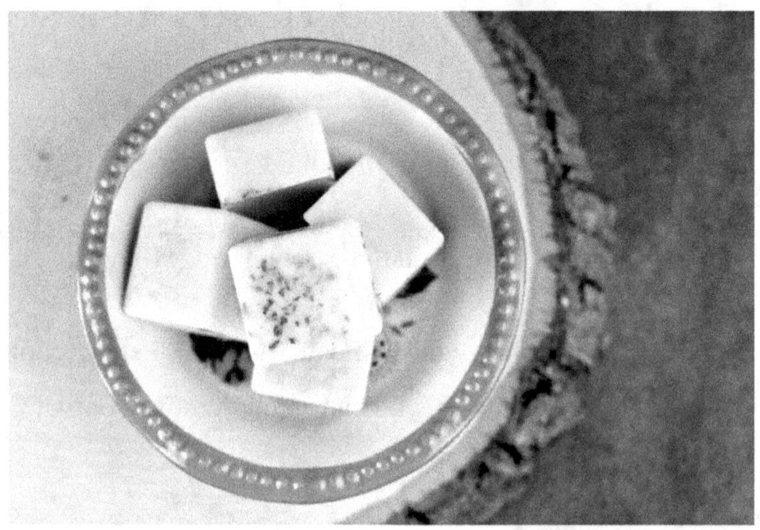

These lotion bars are the perfect thing for your dry skin. The fresh smell of lemon and basil will amaze you. And the best thing is that you can make them quickly. On the other hand, these lotion bars can create the perfect gift too.

Ingredients:

- ¼ cup of coconut oil
- ¼ cup shea butter
- 1 tablespoon grapeseed oil
- 1 tablespoon avocado oil
- ½ tablespoon dried basil

- ½ cup beeswax pastilles

- 15 drops of lemongrass essential oil

- ½ tablespoon dried lemon peel

- 15 drops of basil essential oil

Instructions:

1. Melt the grapeseed oil avocado oil, coconut oil, beeswax and shea butter in a double boiler. Keep to medium heat until everything is melted.

2. Remove from the stove and mix well. Once slightly cooled, add in the essential oils. Mix again.

3. Next, add in the herbs and mix.

4. When everything is combined, pour the liquid into molds. Let them cool and harden.

Conclusion

Once you have checked these easy lotion recipes, you will become a real professional. Whether you choose to prepare them for you, as a gift or plan to sell them, be sure that everyone will love them.

Conscious buyers know about the ingredients of the products that they buy. If you want to be sure that your skin doesn't get exposed to harsh chemicals, these recipes are all that you will ever need.

Proper skincare starts with natural lotions. There are lots of fluffy and whipped lotions that your skin will love. Also, you will find some natural lotion bar recipes that are very convenient for use. It doesn't matter which ones you pick, your skin will experience the benefits for sure.

www.ingramcontent.com/pod-product-compliance
Lightning Source LLC
Chambersburg PA
CBHW061734250726
48657CB00002B/914